# So You Want To Be A Nursing Assistant

Stephen B. Fraser

Copyright © 2013 Fraser Enterprises

Published in the United States of America

ISBN: 1484010175
ISBN-13: 978-1484010174

# DEDICATION

This book is dedicated to all my friends and colleagues that I have worked with over the years. I wouldn't trade all The blood, sweat and tears we have shared together.

# CONTENTS

# PREFACE

So you are sitting there holding this book and thinking to yourself that you want to be a Nurse's Assistant. Years ago when I had considered this career choice I wished that there had been a book like this to read. After working as a CNA (Certified Nurse's Aide) and training and watching a lot of people leave the field. I decided that this was something that I should do. When people think about becoming a Nursing Assistant, they believe that it is an enjoyable job. For myself and a lot of the people I know and work with it is. However it is also a hard job. It means long hours on your feet, demanding patients, documenting everything you do, and often very little thanks. It can be a very rewarding career, and it can also be very taxing career as well.

In the following pages I will give you an  idea of what you can typically expect from a career as a Nursing Assistant. We will cover all aspects of the Nursing Assistants job. I will share my personal experiences as well and colleagues experiences as well. I will finish with some tips and tricks that you will only learn after you have done this job for a while.

Now I can't guarantee that every aspect is in this book. It is however going to be a nice overview of all the things they never teach you in class, and a primer on what it is really like after you start working.

Let me give you a little background about me.  I have been

working in the health care field for eight years. Four in emergency medicine, and four in nursing care/support. I have experience in Trauma, Emergent, Non-Emergent, Geriatric, Long-term, and Short term care. I will not say that I have experienced everything in my career but I have been exposed to a lot in that eight year period. I am certified in three states as a CNA, and have worked as a home health aide as well.

So let's get started…

# WHAT IS A NURSING ASSISTANT

Nursing Assistants are often classified as Unlicensed Assistive Personnel (UAP). This is an umbrella term to describe a job class of paraprofessionals who assist individuals with physical disabilities, mental impairments, and other health care needs with their activities of daily living (ADLs) and provide bedside care. This is all under the supervision of a Registered Nurse, Licensed Practical Nurse or other health care professional. They provide care for patients in hospitals, residents of nursing facilities, clients in private homes, and others in need of their services due to effects of old age or disability.

Nursing Assistants do not hold a license or other mandatory professional requirements for practice. However though many hold various certifications. Often it is required that to work in certain environments you need to be Certified. They are referred to by many titles Nursing Assistant, Nursing Auxiliary, Auxiliary Nurse, Patient Care Assistant, Patient Care Technician, Home Health Aide, Geriatric Aide, Nurse Aide, or Nurse Tech. While they go by many titles for the remainder of the book we will just use the term CNA.

There are some differences in scope of care across UAPs based on title and description. Typically, government certification indicates a more in-depth training and qualification that covers a wider scope of responsibility. These certification exams are distributed by the state. Classes to study for these exams are provided by the American Red

Cross as well as other providers. The courses offered by the American Red Cross encompass all facets that are addressed in the state exams from communication to health terms to sensitivity. CNA's performs everyday living tasks for the elderly, chronically sick, or rehabilitation patients who cannot care for themselves.

CNA's typically can be found working in any number of health care facilities including.

**Urgent Care Center** - a facility or a distinct part of a health care facility which provides preventative, diagnostic, and treatment services to persons who come to the facility to receive services and depart from the facility on the same day.

**Same Day Surgery** - a surgical facility in which ambulatory surgical cases are performed and which is licensed as an ambulatory surgery facility, separate and apart from any other facility license.

**Birth Center** - a health care facility which provides routine prenatal care to low-risk maternity patients or labor and delivery services not requiring surgical intervention.

**Dialysis Center** – a facility that provides dialysis to a patient with end stage renal disease in whom recovery of renal function is not expected.

**Comprehensive Rehabilitation Hospital** - means a facility licensed to provide comprehensive rehabilitation services to patients for the alleviation or amelioration of the disabling effects of illness.

**Hospital** - an facility for the diagnosis, treatment or care of two or more non-related individuals suffering from illness, injury or deformity and where emergency, out-patient, surgical, obstetrical, convalescent or other medical and nursing care is rendered for periods exceeding 24 hours.

**Home Health Agency** - a facility which is licensed to provide preventative, rehabilitative, and therapeutic services to patients in the patient's home or place of residence.

**Hospice** – a program which is licensed to provide palliative services to terminally ill patients in the patients home or place of residence, including medical, nursing, social work, volunteer and counseling services.

**Adult Day Care** - a facility or a distinct part of a facility which is licensed to provide preventive, diagnostic, therapeutic, and rehabilitative services under medical and nursing supervision to meet the needs of functionally impaired adult participants, which does not exceed 12 hours during any calendar day.

**Assisted Living Center** - a facility that is licensed to provide apartment-style housing and congregate dining and to assure that assisted living services are available when needed, to four or more adult persons unrelated to the proprietor. Apartment units offer, at a minimum, one unfurnished room, a private bathroom, a kitchenette, and a lockable door on the unit entrance.

**Skilled Nursing/Nursing Home** - a facility that is licensed to provide health care under medical supervision and continuous nursing care for 24 or more consecutive hours to two or more patients who do not require the degree of care and treatment which a hospital provides and who, because of their physical or mental condition, require continuous nursing care and services above the level of room and board.

**Specialty Hospital** - a hospital which maintains and operates organized facilities and services for the diagnosis, treatment or care of persons suffering from acute illness, injury or deformity.

The type of facility that you work in will determine the amount and types of cares you will provide to patients. In general there are some skills that you will do on a regular basis, and others you will only do only on certain occasions. In all situations you will be working closely with a nurse who is responsible for all cares you provide to a patient. In most facilities you will receive training (also called delegation) to assure that you can effectively provide cares that meet a certain standard of care.

# CERTIFICATION

The question that most people ask is do I need to be certified to work as a Nursing Assistant. The answer is Yes and No, Some states allow people to work as a Nursing Assistant or care givers in certain facilities whether they are certified or not. Typically workers for Home Health Agencies and Assisted Living Centers are not required to be certified. However to work in almost any other type of facility you will need to take a class and get your certification.

The Omnibus Budget Reconciliation Act (OBRA) of 1987 requires Skilled Nursing Facilities (SNFs) and Nursing Facilities (NFs) to use as nurse aides any individuals who have successfully completed a nurse aide training and competency evaluation program (NATCEP) or competency evaluation program (CEP) approved by the State.

Each state must maintain a Registry of all Certified Nursing Assistants (CNAs). This registry contains information on whether an individual has a current CNA certificate. Employers are required to verify currency of a CNAs certificate at the time of employment and upon renewal.

Typically a CNA training program will be a state approved 120 hour course. This includes 80 hours of classroom instruction and 40 hours of clinical instruction. Typically at the end of the class you will take your competency skills exam and written exam. The benefit of clinical instruction is you get to preform skills in an environment with another

CNA. This also gives you a small taste of what daily life is like for a CNA. After clinical instruction some students realize that being a CNA is not really for them and never take the written or skills exam.

What you learn in CNA training becomes just the beginning of the training you will receive. You will also learn the proper way to perform the skills. You will receive Basic Life Support (BLS) training. Also known as CPR. Unfortunately in this career you will use this training several times.

After you complete your CNA class and get your certification from the state in which you wish to work in you will now have enough skills to get a job in an Assisted Living Center, or Skilled Nursing Facility. If your dreams are to work in a Hospital or other Facility. You will want to gain more skills and training. But you will also want to hone your patient care skills as well.

Based on where you want to work you will want to get additional training. No one can grantee that just because you have additional skills or training that you will get employed, but in my experience it never hurts. Anything that you can use to make yourself more marketable is always a good idea.

I will list some additional training you might wish to get and the reason it is helpful.


**Assistance with Medications** – In Assisted Living Centers you will be asked to assist residents with their medications. This is also helpful in some Home Health Agencies that allow staff to assist with medications.

**ACLS (Advanced Cardiac Life Support)** – You will learn advanced skills that will come in handy when working in Cardiac departments and Emergency Rooms.

**ECG Interpretation** – Even though most Hospitals have Monitor Technicians this is still a good skill to have.

**Mental Illness Training** – Since you may on occasion have to work with patients with Mental illness this is a necessity.

**Dementia and Alzheimer's Training** – Essential if you are going to be working with the Elderly or the Geriatric community.

This is just a short list anything that you see that can give you more knowledge or can make it easier to do your job will be invaluable. Unfortunately throughout your career you will also need Continuing Education Units (CEU's) as well. These trainings will often fill those CEU credits too.

# WHAT DOES A CNA DO

As we have already said CNA stands for Certified Nurse's Assistant. Although sometimes throughout your career you will feel like it stands for Certified Nurse's whipping boy, Certified Mushroom, and Certified Butt Wiper. Being a CNA can be a very rewarding and fulfilling career. However even rewarding careers have their drawbacks.

In a typical day your duties as a CNA will encompass most of the following.

- Observing, documenting and reporting clinical and treatment information, including patients' behavioral changes
- Assisting with range of motion exercises
- Taking and recording blood pressure, temperature, pulse, respiration, and bodyweight
- Assisting with ambulating and mobilization of patients
- Collecting specimens for required medical tests
- Providing emotional and support services to patients, their families and other caregivers
- Assisting with personal hygiene
- Assisting with meal preparation, grocery shopping, dietary planning, and food and fluid intake.

In a typical day you may have to bathe a patient, dress them, feed them and change them. You may also have to do laundry, change linens, and perform housekeeping.  Depending on where you are working you may be responsible for between one to twelve patients (sometimes more).  You may have to deal with Colostomies and/or Catheters. You will become very familiar with bodily waste.  You will collect specimens for testing. In between all of that you will also asked to do any number of other things that your nurse will ask you to do.

You will be exposed to infectious materials and waste.  It will ultimately be your responsibility to make sure you take the appropriate precautions when dealing with these items.  Several peoples careers have been impacted because they contracted something from someone else simply because they didn't follow basic precautions. That is why it is always important to remember your training and not get caught up in a rush just to save time.

Also in the course of your day you are going to have a lot of interaction with your patients.  It is how you interact with your patients that is going to be the most important part of your job.  Often they may be confused, bored, depressed, or lonely.  Often they are all of the above at the same time.  Think about what it would be like if you were in their place.  You  can easily see how your attitude and manner can affect the situation.

At the end of your day you will document everything you did over the course of your shift and give report to the CNA that will be relieving you. Your documentation should only contain facts about what you did, or did not do and the reason why.  Afterwards you get to go home and relax and prepare to do it all over again the next day.

Caring for people is in every sense of the term is what you will do every day. My personal belief is you can't care for someone without caring for them. That being said I approach my job from a different position than most people. Every patient I interact with I treat as if they were my Mother, Father, Grandparent, Child, or Spouse. However when working in long term care you often build relationships with your patients. The drawback is when they pass on you end up going through the grief process just as if they were your own family. In my experience dealing with death never gets any easier no matter how often it happens. Everybody deals with death in different ways unfortunately there are no tips I can offer to help you with that aspect of this job.

# WHAT DOES A CNA GET PAID

In a quick answer to that question is <u>Not Nearly Enough</u>. However it is hard to place an actual figure on it because every part of the country is different. Since CNA's typically earn an hourly wage rather than an annual salary, your pay will fluctuate depending on whether you take a few hours here and there, or work full time. According to the Bureau of Labor Statistics, the median wage for CNAs was $11.63/ Hr. in May 2011. The median wage for Home Health Aides: $9.91/ Hr. in May 2011.

This does not mean that you will be paid that much a lot of it depends on where you are working. Typically it goes like this Home Health Aides are paid the lowest. Then its followed by CNA's in Assisted Living Centers or Adult Daycare Centers. Followed with Hospice. Then comes Skilled Nursing Centers and Nursing Homes. Then Hospitals and Advanced Care Centers.

| Place of Work | Pay rate (per hour) |
|---|---|
| Home Health Aide | $9.00 |
| Assisted Living / Adult Daycare | $9.50 |
| Hospice | $10.00 |
| Skilled Nursing / Nursing Home | $10.50 |
| Hospital / Advanced Care | $12.00 – $13.00 |

Table 1 Based on starting wages for the State of Idaho

As you can see the State of Idaho is below the Bureau of Labor Statistics median wage. This doesn't take into account benefits and other compensation such as tuition assistance, health insurance, uniform allowance, etc. It is also important to state that CNA's are usually considered an entry level position. This is typically because most CNA's continue on with their schooling or training to become Nurses or other professionals in the medical field. That is not to say that you won't meet CNA's that have decided to make this their career field. I know a lot of career care givers and CNA's.

# THE BASICS

At this point if you are still reading this you have decided that this is a career you are interested in pursuing, or that you have resigned yourself to doing till you get done with schooling, in either case congratulations. I am going to break this chapter up into segments that will cover things you will want to know prior to going to work in this exciting field.

## Uniforms

First things first is clothing. Before we talk about anything else lets discuss footwear. Shoes are quickly going to be the most important thing you buy. You need to consider that you will be on your feet at least 8 hours or as long as 12 hours. Depending on your shift schedule you may only get a 30 minute lunch break and one or two 10 minutes breaks. There may be periods where you are able to sit down. However in my experience these have been few and far between. As a result your feet take the most abuse from this type of work.

When you think about shoes it is important to think about the fact that you are not going to wear these anywhere else but at work. The reason being is that you may get things on them that you don't want to share with others outside of work. (i.e. vomit, blood, urine and fecal material) I can't stress enough especially for women. Don't get concerned with wearing cute shoes.

When buying shoes the primary concerns are comfort and support. You will want to buy a shoe that is close-toed, with good arch support and a moderate amount of cushioning in the foot bed. Some people prefer to buy running shoes because of their cushioning. I prefer to buy shoes that have a cork or air cell foot bed. The reason being is cork and air cell foot beds conform to the shape of your foot and distribute the shock across the entire foot making walking less taxing on your feet. You should consider lace up shoes as opposed to slip-on shoes. I try to tell people to stay away from white colored shoes as well for obvious reasons. You will also want a non-skid sole and a non-marking sole will be appreciated by the housekeeping staff too.

I suggest that you try on your shoes before you buy them walk around the store and see how they feel. You will sometimes see Scrub supply stores that sell shoes that are antimicrobial or bio-hazard resistant. This is nice but often unneeded. In my experience anything I have gotten on my shoes can be wiped off and then treated with a sanitizing chemical spray. Try to buy two pairs of shoes and alternate between them. Wearing one pair one day and another pair the next will not only slow shoe breakdown but will also spare your feet.

Scrubs are the generally accepted uniform for CNA's. Some home health agencies may allow you to wear normal clothes, but in almost all facilities scrubs will be the required attire. Hopefully you live in an area where you have a store that sells scrubs and other nursing equipment. This will be the preferred place to purchase your scrubs. During schooling you will probably be required to where a particular color of scrubs for your clinicals. After that you will probably be able to wear just about what ever color you wish. I have heard of some employers wanting CNA's wear a particular color or colors only. This is typically few and far between.

There is currently approximately 30-40 different companies that make scrubs. This is nice because it means there are a lot of styles to choose from. Just like any other clothing you will be able to find a style that works for you. There are different pocket styles, top, and bottom styles to choose from. For instance you may find that you prefer an elastic waist pant as opposed to a tie waist pant. You may find you like a certain pocket configuration than another. You can also choose from many options for tops as well.

You will want to have at least one top and bottom for each day or shift you work. For example if you work a 4-2 rotation (4 days on, 2 days off) you would want five tops and bottoms. Also you may find that you want a couple of undershirts for added warmth during cold weather. As far as undershirts I prefer Under Armour© Compression t-shirts and Long sleeve mock turtlenecks. Mostly due to their moisture wicking ability.

You will want to wear a clean pair of scrubs for each shift and will want to wash your scrubs separately from your normal every day wear clothes or your families clothes. The best way to think of it is anything you pick up on your clothes at work you don't want to share with your family. Because of this constant wash and wear cycle do not be surprised if your scrubs are wearing out faster than you expected. It is an unfortunate fact of working in the medical field.

Finally you will want to wear foundation garments under your scrubs. Scrubs are made loose fitting for a reason, and as a result certain movements may reveal more than you intend. Once you find a style of scrubs you like you will likely want to continually wear them. Usually you can take the style number off the tag and purchase them online and save some money.

## Equipment

Typically as a CNA there will be no equipment that you will need to purchase. That being said there is a few things that you may want to consider purchasing for your own use. Most every place you will work will have a set of vitals equipment for you to use. In my experience this equipment is used by all employees and often not cleaned after it is used. As far as things like pulse oximeters and BP cuffs this is not a huge problem. However when you are talking about Stethoscopes it does tend to be more of an issue. More so than just the hygiene issues there is the fact that Stethoscopes that are purchased for floor use are usually low quality and difficult to hear through. My personal suggestion is to purchase at a minimum a Stethoscope and BP cuff.

While we are on the subject of stethoscopes keep in mind that the higher the price the better the quality. Personally I own the Littmann® Master Classic II. I have had this over 4 years and it works flawlessly, Also replacement parts can be purchased from Littmann. There are several different types of Stethoscopes that are available out there all have different acoustic levels and will enable you to hear different sounds. I personally have diminished hearing so I specifically chose the Master Classic II for its superior sound quality. Think of this as an investment in your profession. I would rather buy a $200 stethoscope once every 5-7 years than a $20 one every year.

If you are going to purchase your own Stethoscope remember to take care of it. At the end of your shift take a alcohol swap and wipe it down from head to the tubing and the ear pieces. This will be sufficient to kill most microorganisms on it as well as make it sanitary for the patient as well. Also invest in a name tag for your stethoscope. It diminishes the chance of losing it or having it stolen.

There is other equipment that you may find useful to have. But each person is different. So I will leave that up to you. Other than my own Stethoscope, BP cuff, and watch. I carry a pair of bandage scissors and a pen light. The bandage scissors are useful for cutting gauze or tape for a nurse when you are assisting them (or when they forget to bring their own). A pen light is useful when entering a dark room with a sleeping patient to read the Oxygen flow or other things without having to turn on the overhead light and waking them up.

Finally the most important thing every CNA should own and have with them every shift is a watch. I know this sounds dumb but you need a watch with a second hand. Do not buy a digital one. You will need the second hand when doing a pulse rate or respiratory rate. Since these are done by observing in relation to a minute of time. Since most CNA's in an effort to save time will count for 20 seconds and multiply the result by 3, or count for 30 seconds and multiply by 2. A second hand is definitely needed. Personally I prefer a watch with dual displays. It has a watch face with hands and then a smaller digital window that allows me set it to 24-hour time (also referred to as Military time). This makes it easier when doing documentation since most facilities prefer that documentation be done in 24-hour time.

One final thing to mention about equipment and uniforms. Since the likely hood is that you are going to be paying for these out of your own pocket. Keep all your receipts for tax purposes. At the end of the year you will be able to get a credit on your taxes for all equipment you purchase for use in your job. This includes all equipment, uniforms, Shoes, etc.

## Immunizations

Because of the nature of the environment and the patients you are working with you will come in contact with some infectious diseases. Most employers will ask you if you have had certain immunizations. If you haven't they may offer you to get them. Certain immunizations like Hepatitis B, you will definitely want to get because of how easily it can be transmitted. However you always have the right to refuse them for personal or religious reasons. You may also need to get a current TB test. Usually in the fall your employer may offer the Influenza (Flu) shot. Since your patients may have it or you may get it outside of work. You should consider getting the shot. Missing work due to the flu is often hard on the paycheck, I would rather have to miss one day as opposed to three or four days.

Always keep records of your Immunizations and TB tests. This saves time later when you change employers or in the unfortunate case where you are exposed to something. Having this information makes it easier for everyone involved in either situation.

## Odors and Smells

You will quickly learn that this is a very odiferous profession. You will find that there are smells that are helpful and others that are not. I can tell you if a patient has a UTI or CDIF simply by smell. Now I don't make a habit of smelling urine or feces but you will undoubtedly smell it regardless. If you have problems with odors and smells there are a few options. First some might tell you to just breathe through your mouth.

This is a bad idea  for one simple reason.  If you don't want to smell it you definitely don't want to taste it.  If you are breathing through your mouth you will definitely taste it.  A second option that you can employ is to put a little Vicks® inside your nostrils before shift and after breaks. I have done this and found it does work  quite well but overpowering odors still get through.  The third and as I have found the most effective is to just ignore the odor since the human body can quickly acclimate to smells. The odor usually only bothers you for only a few seconds. If you control your breathing you will find you will not notice the smell as mush or even at all.  Since the body's first reaction to a repulsive smell is to  move away from an offensive odor or stop breathing temporarily. When you take that next breath the odor is even more overwhelming. With practice you can continue to breath normally and the odor will quickly become unnoticeable.  This is the same reason why when you use an air freshener you only smell it for a few moments and then no longer notice it.

You may find that there are some odors you cannot get past. For me that happens to be the smell of Cancer.  Anyone who has been on the oncology ward knows what that smell is.  No matter how much I try I just can't get past that smell.  You may find that certain smells will be like that for you as well.

**Stress**

It is just a part of the job.  Yes it is true that every job brings stress. Finding how you mitigate and reduce your stress is the most important thing you can do. Some people you work with will have low stress tolerances.  Others will seem like they are not bothered by it at all.

Everybody de-stresses differently, some people smoke, drink, or just need to walk away for a few minutes. Knowing your triggers and how to de-stress will be paramount to your job performance. Knowing when you need to step away is important, but so is knowing that you may not be able to when you need too. Also no employer is going to be happy if you need 30 smoke breaks every day just to de-stress. Look for effective ways to release your stress outside of work. Get away from the facility, go for a run, play with your dog. Whatever it is make it a part of your daily work routine. In the end you will be happier and healthier.

**Physical Fitness**

I won't lie this is a very physically demanding job. The fact that you are on your feet for 90% of your shift is hard enough on your body. When you throw in the constant lifting, bending, turning, carrying, and walking. It quickly becomes very taxing to your physicality. There is an old saying that says "If you have a good back going into this job you won't have one when you come out." Sadly there is some truth to it. You will need to be aware that you using proper body mechanics when lifting and moving patients. If you have access to a gym use it and exercise. You don't have to be lifting weights and getting buffed out but conditioning and stamina with be very beneficial in your work. The other benefit to working out is it gives you a great way to alleviate stress.

Maintaining a healthy and physically fit body is essential for two very important reasons. First if and when you get injured whether it is on the job or off you will heal faster. Secondly you will find that often you may have to deal with two-person assists by yourself. Being physically strong enough to work with a patient will become essential in your job.

# I'M CERTIFIED NOW WHAT

Congratulations you passed your skills evaluation and written test, and now you have your Nursing Assistant Certification. First remember this is not a license. This is a certification. What's the difference? Simple a license is often associated with schooling (one to two years) a degree (A.A. or A.A.S.) and usually includes a component of Clinical hours. The testing requirements afterwards are more in-depth as well. Is it a major issue if you refer to it as a license. In short no, but I have seen Nurses and others get upset when people have called it that.

Your next step is to go find a job in your new career field. Usually about a week after you finish your testing you should receive your certification from the state that you are certified in. It is not essential that you have this prior to looking for a job but it does make it easier since you can put your certification number on the application. This allows the employer to look you up and verify your certification prior to interviewing you. Now if you live on the border of one state and another you can reciprocate your certification to another state. This allows you to work in another state. Most states have rules the require that CNA's must be certified in their state of employment. This is the reason for why I am certified in three states. Each state will have its own rules as to what a CNA can do, and not do. They will sometimes differ greatly between states. Some states may even require you to take additional training that you will need to show proof of before reciprocating your certification.

You will find that most often the jobs open to you as a new CNA will be in Home Health Care, Assisted Living, and Skilled Nursing Facilities. This is not to say that you cannot get employed at a Hospital or Advanced Care Facility. It is just that positions in Hospitals often want to see that CNA's have at a minimum of a year of experience in patient care and duties of a CNA. However there is always the exception and as everyone knows if you know the right people you can sometimes benefit from those relationships.

When you get your interview dress professionally. Make sure your hair is combed and that you are presentable. Bring at least two copies of your resume, certification, and any other documents. Place them in groups with your Resume on top, followed by your state CNA Certification or Certification card. Then place your other documents such as your CPR card, and any other training certificates. (Alzheimer's and Dementia Training, Medication Assistance, etc.) Make sure you carry them in a folder to protect them and keep them looking good. Never carry your original documents to an interview. Always make copies of your originals and then place them in a safe place. Always use photocopies to carry with you. When they ask for them you can hand them to them and they keep them for their records. Later in your career you will want to add letters of recommendations to your document pack. These should always be from Nurse's you have worked with and who can accurately evaluate your skills.

# LESSONS LEARNED

In this just a final chapter I am going to cover a few things that I have learned over the years working as a CNA.

Find a bag that you are comfortable with to carry your Stethoscope and other gear you take and use at work. It can be a fanny pack or a small backpack.

It is always a good idea to carry a spare pair of scrubs to work with you. Several times because of the nature of the job you will either get something on your scrubs that you don't want to wear all shift and will want to change or you might have a wardrobe malfunction and need to change your scrubs because of it.

Death is inevitable especially when working with the elderly. It happens and it is part of life. You will form attachments to your residents and when they pass it will be hard. Just understand that it is just part of healing.

You will not get along with every one of your co-workers all the time. Remember that you are there for your patients. If you simply can't get along with a co-worker talk to your supervisor.

Leave your work at work. Never talk to anyone outside of work about your patients or their status. First off it is a major HIPAA violation and it is highly unprofessional.

A smile can defuse even the most upset resident. Always maintain eye contact and smile it will make your job easier.

Your nurse is your biggest ally. When they ask you to do something you don't know how to do. Tell them you don't know how to do that or that you have never been shown how to do it. If they have time they will show you and then the next time they will feel comfortable in your abilities.

Never attempt to do a task you have never performed before. I can grantee it will be a learning experience for you and not in a good way.

Always ask questions even if you think it is a stupid one. People would rather you ask questions than do something wrong.

CPR is an essential skill learn to do it correctly. Be prepared for when the time comes it will feel and sound completely different then the manikin you train on.

Use all your abilities. I mentioned before that I can tell with about 95% accuracy if a patient has a UTI, or C-Diff by the smell. Also if it doesn't look like it should normally that is something you need to convey to the Nurse.

You spend most of your time with the patient. Observe and report what doesn't seem right, or is unusual. CNA's will often see the subtle changes that others may miss.

Time management is a key skill to learn if you don't you will be behind every day and go home tired night.

Realize that you not only care for you patients but their family as well.

Smartphones are a great tool. Some employers may allow you to carry one during work. There are several apps for both iPhone and Android that can help with everything from Dosage Calculations to Drug Identification and everything in between. These will prove invaluable.

# ABOUT THE AUTHOR

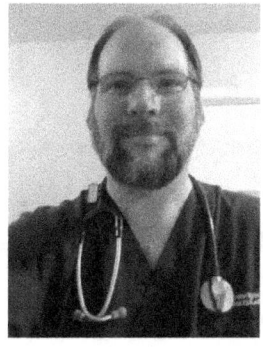

Stephen B. Fraser (1971- ) was born in Sacramento, California. While growing up in North Idaho and Western Montana he learned to appreciate the outdoors and the naturalist lifestyle. He is a confirmed realist, and student of human nature. He has written several short stories under a couple of pen names. His first book was released in Feb 2012 under his own name. He completed his second book in October and revised and re-released his first book in November. Stephen currently resides in beautiful North Idaho with his dog Ollie where he enjoys camping, fishing, and continues to work in the Healthcare field. When he is not writing he is pursuing his other interests.

You can contact Stephen at the following:

stephenbfraser.com

Twitter @stephenbfraser

## Other Books by Stephen B. Fraser

Men: The Handbook

Politics 101

www.ingramcontent.com/pod-product-compliance
Lightning Source LLC
Chambersburg PA
CBHW070526290526
45790CB00003B/1313